DEPRESSION
Drowning In Air

A Young Man's Staggering Journey From Hopeless To Hopeful

A.J. REIMER

Depression: Drowning In Air – A Young Man's Staggering Journey From Hopeless To Hopeful Copyright © 2014 by Jacob Reimer.

All rights reserved. No part of this book may be reproduced in any form without permission in writing from the author. Reviewers may quote brief passages in reviews.

Disclaimer

No part of this publication may be reproduced or transmitted in any form or by any means, mechanical or electronic, including photocopying or recording, or by any information storage and retrieval system, or transmitted by email without permission in writing from the publisher.

While all attempts have been made to verify the information provided in this publication, neither the author nor the publisher assumes any responsibility for errors, omissions, or contrary interpretations of the subject matter herein.

This book is for entertainment purposes only. The views expressed are those of the author alone, and should not be taken as expert instruction or commands. The reader is responsible for his or her own actions.

Adherence to all applicable laws and regulations, including international, federal, state, and local governing professional licensing, business practices, advertising, and all other aspects of doing business in the US, Canada, or any other jurisdiction is the sole responsibility of the purchaser or reader.

Neither the author nor the publisher assumes any responsibility or liability whatsoever on the behalf of the purchaser or reader of these materials.

Any perceived slight of any individual or organization is purely unintentional.

WHO I AM, AND WHY I WROTE THIS BOOK

You could say I'm nobody. I have no degree. I'm not a licensed professional. I'm not a doctor—I don't even play one on TV.

What I do have is my experience. I've been through anxiety and depression. I've hit rock bottom, shattering so hard that I thought I could never be put back together. I lay there, wounded, for years, only to find a sense of motivation from within that I didn't know existed—a resilience in my very being that wouldn't allow me to give up without a fight. I patched my wounds, staggered to my feet, and stood tall for the world—and myself—to see. Then I took my first step towards freedom.

Overcoming depression isn't something that happens overnight. It's a journey. By showing you my journey, I want to provide you with a sense of hope. I want to equip you with the tools necessary to make your own journey, and guide you towards the first step.

I've experienced and suffered more than others, but I believe that all the troubles I've gone through have happened for a reason. I believe that they strengthened, challenged, and molded me into the man I am today. That's something I would never change.

I'm eager to share what I've learned along the way, so you can benefit from my struggles, too. My purpose in writing this book is to be a beacon of hope to those still stuck in the storm. I want you to know that you are not alone. There is light at the end of the tunnel.

That doesn't mean it's easy. Crap happens, and life is full of difficulties that we never could have seen coming. Just know that, even though life happens to us all, there is hope. There is an entire community of people behind you. There are support systems and groups longing to love and cherish you for who YOU are right now. Above all else, there's a strength inside of you that you don't yet know exists. With this book, I want to show it you.

I wrote this book to give you the same guidance and advice that helped me immensely during my own journey. It contains no fluff or hype, just the truth about my journey, my struggles, and what I did to come out stronger on the other side.

TABLE OF CONTENTS

INTRODUCTION I

PROLOGUE: Facing My Demons 1

PART I: Everything Changed 5

PART II: Abused 29

PART III: Breaking Point 43

PART IV: Recovery 61

PART V: Advice For Others 73

PART VI: How To Enjoy Life Again 109

ABOUT AUTHOR 129

ACKNOWLEDGEMENTS 131

INTRODUCTION

Welcome to *"Depression: My Battle - A Young Man's Staggering Journey From Hopeless To Hopeful."*

I want to start off by thanking you for purchasing this book! It was not an easy one to write. However, I hope that by sharing my experiences and the tools and resources I used to overcome them, I may be able to help someone else who is still struggling through their journey.

Depression has definitely become more recognized in recent years in general society. But that doesn't mean it's widely accepted, understood, or properly dealt with. I believe that one of the best ways to improve this is through education, especially through hearing from people who are brave enough to share their stories. That is my intention with this book: to use my story to help you understand depression and learn how you can help yourself if you're struggling.

In this book, I share my secrets and show you some of the darkest times of my life. It's been hard to write about these times, but above all, I want you to know that you're not alone. I got through my dark times, and with the right information and help, so can you.

It is not my objective to sugarcoat anything, nor to give you some "quick fix" solution. There is no quick fix for depression, and those who say there is obviously have never truly experienced it for themselves.

What I am going to do is take you along on my journey—sharing, spilling, and explaining it as best I can. In addition, I will reveal how I personally found healing and hope. This is no proven step-by-step system, just my real experiences.

Life is hard and littered with challenges. Yet, if we can learn to properly cope with these challenges, life can became an incredibly wondrous gift, overflowing with joy, love, and discovery.

It's not always easy, but it *is* possible. With the right support system and some courage and perseverance, I know that you can make it through this and become a stronger person because of it.

Thank you again for your purchase, and I truly

DROWNING IN AIR

hope you enjoy my book!

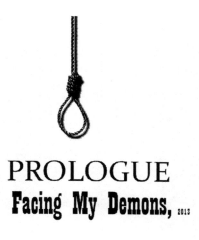

PROLOGUE
Facing My Demons, 2013

I've finally had enough. The frustration of feeling trapped inside the cell of my hopeless existence has become too much to bear. I feel like a massive bundle of ice and snow teetering on the edge of a cliff, with only a thin branch keeping me from my inevitable destruction.

I hate my life, my friends, and my family. Above all, I hate myself.

I flee to my downstairs bathroom, the only room with a lock, and pace back and forth. My mind is racing, yet I'm not really thinking.

"This is ridiculous," I mutter to myself.

I can't understand how things could have gotten to this point. It seems like only yesterday that I was a happy child, cheerfully playing in my world of ignorance. Yet those days are long gone, along with my sanity.

How I long for just a moment's peace! I feel like I haven't been able to breathe for...days? weeks? months? I can't even remember. The mere thought of peace and quiet seems so foreign to my mind, I don't even remember what it felt like. I would give anything for just a moment's rest.

My eyes are wide, jaw clenched shut. My primal instincts take over, as if they can predict the doom to come.

My head moves in irregular patterns, which I have little control over, and I don't care why.

I'm fighting my inner demons... and I'm losing.

Like an avalanche, my rage is suddenly released with an amount of force and energy I didn't know I was capable of holding. Time seems to slow down as my fist travels through the air and continues directly through the beige bathroom wall.

I stand in disbelief, frozen in fear of what I have just done.

I return to my senses and take stock of my surroundings. My fist, still embedded in the wall, is dripping with blood. More blood drips down the wall toward my bare toes.

How could I have lost control like that?

Suddenly, I'm struck with great remorse. It hits me like a ton of bricks, knocking me down from my adrenaline high. I'm petrified of the punishment that awaits me for my recklessness.

I consider trying to explain, but I know it won't do any good. I take a deep breath and hold it, then release it, along with all the tension in my body. I know what I have to do.

"This is it," I say aloud for only myself to hear. "I'm done."

I've considered suicide before, but this time is different. All the other times, I saw a way out—something I could do to make life a little better. This time, I see no way out, no help, and no hope. The relentless internal struggle is far beyond unbearable, and I no longer have the strength to fight it.

I stand up, calmly and steadily making my way from the bathroom toward my bedroom. I'm not nervous or scared... just tired.

My journey will soon be over, and along with it, my suffering.

How did I ever get to this point?

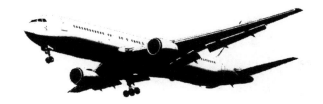

PART I
Everything Changed

"You can never truly appreciate that which you have never truly lost."

Thailand, 2005

My story begins in the summer of 2005, when my parents were offered the opportunity to move to Thailand for missions work. Up to this point, I had grown up in British Columbia, but long-time family friends of ours were running a missionary outreach in Chon Buri. They wanted our help in establishing an orphanage for children who had contracted HIV or AIDS. These children were born with the virus, carried by their mothers. The children had little hope and little help, and most of them felt completely worthless.

With the devastation of the tragic 2004 tsunami that struck most of Southeast Asia still fresh in our minds, we decided to go on a short one-month scouting trip to get a feel for the country and to help with the tsunami relief efforts.

Tsunami

When we arrived for our scouting trip, we became immersed in the epic landscape, utterly torn apart by the fury of Mother Nature. The entire experience was completely surreal.

I still remember walking on a cement pathway, seemingly in the middle of nowhere. To my left was a barren wasteland of debris as far as the eye could see. It continued for another 200 yards or so on my right, only yielding at the base of a massive mountain. Amazingly, a few homes built entirely of concrete had survived the ordeal. But even for these lucky few, though the foundations and walls still stood, everything inside was completely destroyed, including all the families' belongings.

One of these homes in particular stood out to me. What made it stand out was a massive fishing boat pressed up against the front of the house. Like an extremely large arrowhead, the nose of the ship was perfectly in line to split the house in half.

We also got the opportunity to speak with the owner of the home, who happened to be inside it when the tsunami hit. He said he was awoken from a dead sleep by a loud thumping noise. He thought someone was pounding on the front door, so he roused himself from his bed on the second floor and opened the window to see who it was. However, instead of a person, he was stunned to find the front of a massive fishing vessel staring him in the face. The man later showed us the stain that the water had left on his home. It turned out to measure around eight feet high, and we were over a half mile inland.

Another sight that stuck in my mind was an even larger steel military boat that was pressed up against the side of the mountain 200 yards to my right. I stared at it with dumbfounded amazement, wondering how something so massive could have been placed so elegantly on the mountainside. I thought that it must have been built right where it lay, as I could see no other way that something so large and mighty could have ended up where it was. I ended up asking a rather dumb question to our Thai guide, saying, "Where did that ship come from?"

He smiled at me, since the answer was quite obvious, and said, "The ocean carried it there."

Undeterred by the reply to my first foolish question, my uncanny wit mustered up the brilliant response of, "But where is the ocean?"

He only laughed and pointed to my left, in the direction of the wasteland. He said, "You see those palm trees?"

I had to squint, but now that I knew what to look for, I could spot them on the horizon. I nodded.

"Well, that is the shoreline. The water carried the ship all the way there and was only stopped by the mountain."

It was hard to fathom. However, I knew there was no other explanation that could account for the massive ship ending up where it lay. In that moment, I gained a newfound respect for the power of nature. It both amazed and terrified me.

Leaving Home

A few months after our short adventure ended, my parents made the bold decision to uproot our family and move to Thailand for a one-year term.

My sister, who is nearly three years my elder, was ecstatic. She felt a pull toward adventure and deeply desired the thrill of experiencing a new culture. I, on the other hand, did not. Everything I had ever known was in North America. I was born in Fresno, California, and I had lived there for the first four years of my life. After that, my family moved to beautiful British Columbia, and it was there where I grew up.

All of my friends and all of my passions were in British Columbia: my grandparents, my home, my soccer team, everything. How could I leave it all behind? You can't just pack up your life in a box and take it with you. Some things would never be the same, for example, my soccer career. I was playing on the highest-level soccer team I could for my age group, and I had been training with the same group of guys since I was six years old. Leaving now meant falling behind and eventually being replaced. At the fragile age of eleven, this was extremely hard to swallow.

I protested and complained all I could, but ultimately my concerns fell on deaf ears. By the summer of 2006, we were off to our new home.

The fact that my objections made no difference in the final outcome hurt me. I had no say in the decision. I felt like my family had betrayed me and my voice had gone unheard. Of course, I was being quite selfish by not also taking into account the needs and desires of the rest of my family, but needless to say, I felt abandoned.

Hospitalized

After the first few months of adjusting to my new life, things slowly turned from bad to worse. I had become withdrawn from my family, and I spent much of my time alone. Looking back on it now, I was already showing signs of clinical depression, but I had no way of knowing that then.

To make things worse, I got sick. One thing you need to understand about living overseas is the sickness that you will inevitably encounter. The simple flu viruses that we deal with here are nothing compared to the viruses that go around in third-world countries. Once flu season arrives, it's like a cat-and-mouse game, except the mouse is stuck in a mousetrap and the cat has 10 buddies on his side. You basically just wait for your turn and hope that it isn't *too* bad.

I already had an immense aversion to throwing up, so when I got my first taste of third-world flu, I did not take it well. It hit me so hard that I actually had to be hospitalized overnight due to the large amounts of fluid that I had lost and my inability to retain anything. When I got home from the hospital, I made it a mission of mine to NEVER have that experience again. To my dismay, this lofty goal was completely out of my reach.

A new form of the flu was already going around within the same year, and I was adamant that I was not going to get it! I did everything in my power to stay healthy, from avoiding those who had come in contact with it to always washing my hands. I also started to take vitamins and supplements that support immune health to give myself a fighting chance. After nearly everyone I knew had caught the bug, I felt victorious. I had accomplished my goal and was going to stay free from the agonizing terror that I dreaded... or so I thought.

Not even a week after I celebrated my success, I caught the flu again. Unfortunately, since I was nearly the last person to catch it, I got it far worse because the virus had had time to mutate and gain more strength as it cycled through others. After one of the worst nights of my life, I was rushed to the hospital with a resting heartbeat of around 180. To give you some context, my normal resting heartbeat is around 45-60 and my heartbeat during intense exercise normally doesn't surpass 160-170. So when my heartbeat was in the 180s as I practiced the rigorous exercise of lying in the fetal position, the doctors were quite worried. They told my mother they were concerned about a potential heart attack, and therefore they wanted me to stay for a few nights so that they could monitor my progress.

If you thought it couldn't get any worse after I left the hospital, then you thought wrong. My parents knew that I had developed a serious anxiety disorder and was on the verge of insanity. I couldn't mentally handle getting sick again. So, in an attempt to give me immunity to the disease, they took me to get a flu shot. Unfortunately for me however, I ended up getting the shot too soon after my departure from the hospital. My body had not yet recovered enough to handle it. I ended up getting my third case of the flu in a year, and again had to be hospitalized overnight.

Not only was I in a place where I didn't want to be, but now I couldn't stop getting sick and throwing up, something I already hated more than the average person. Through this flu experience, I developed a severe anxiety disorder. I began to have frequent, intense panic attacks on a regular basis. In addition, I slipped into full-blown depression, and I virtually stopped living.

Panic Attacks

After that, I became extremely paranoid about the state of my health. I was constantly aware of everything my stomach was doing.

I began to have severe panic attacks on a daily basis. Every day, I thought I was getting the flu. It consumed me and controlled my life. Every time, my parents would tell me that I was simply having another panic attack, and that I wasn't really sick. However, it made no difference. Every attack felt different to me, and I was always convinced that *this* would be the time when I actually got sick. I was terrified that if I ever let my guard down, that would be the time I got sick. Therefore, I lived in constant fear, always scared that today could be the day when I would be sick again.

I began to lose the ability to sleep regularly, as most of these attacks occurred at night. A few months after the panic attacks, I began to get daily stomachaches that would last throughout the entire day. I stopped going out of the house and virtually locked myself in my room. I'm still not sure whether I was trying to stay away from the world, or whether I wanted the world to stay away from me. I was so angry, yet so afraid. My mind was constantly racing, and it began to wear me out.

At this point, I felt as though I had hit rock bottom. I was in a country I didn't like, with people I didn't know, stuck in a family who (I thought) hated me, and I was constantly feeling sick. I officially entered a state of severe depression. Life became rather meaningless. It felt more like a chore to wake up every morning, and I always dreaded the day to follow.

Anyone who has ever been depressed can understand this, though that certainly doesn't make it any easier. Just know that, if you feel this way, you are not alone. There are others who feel the exact same way, and best of all, there is help! I'll explain this in much better detail in the last chapter. So, if you *are* feeling hopeless and don't know what to do, please skip to there **right now**! The whole point of this book is to help others and share what I've learned. So please, if you are anything less than happy, skip to the final chapters, and learn how to finally get the healing you deserve! You can always come back to this point to continue with my story.

Lost Hope

As my panic attacks destroyed my ability to sleep and participate in life, I lost the will to live. In turn, I lost the ability to care about my own well being. I even contemplated suicide. Though my thoughts never materialized into actions, I honestly didn't care if anything happened to me. I decided that I no longer valued the life I had been given. Therefore, I did not fear death, nor try to avoid it. When you no longer fear death, life can become quite a hazardous place. I wasn't going to take my life, but I figured if I died in some kind of freak accident while doing something crazy, then it must have been meant to be.

I avoided dabbling with severely addictive behaviors, such as drinking, experimenting with different drugs, or enjoying the intimate company of women. Instead, I became an adrenaline junkie. The only way I could feel *free* was to perform terrifying and downright idiotic stunts. I began practicing Parkour and often took things to an extremely unsafe level. I got my "high" from literally being high: balancing my body over ledges multiple stories above the concrete below, climbing up billboards and water towers, and walking on the rooftop edges of ten-story buildings.

No matter how dangerous or terrifying the situation I put myself in, I still managed to find beauty in it. There was something serene about being up high, away from everything—only me, the cool air, and the world below. It gave me a sense of freedom and was my form of escape. I guess it allowed me to exit my world for brief stretches of time, and it gave me time to think and recharge. It also helped me gain perspective by allowing me to witness how truly small I am in comparison to the world around me. If I could somehow convince myself that I was small, then maybe I could convince myself that my problems were small, too.

Under Pressure

In addition to the stomach problems, I was also subjected to an onslaught of unfair treatment by the missions director. She had been a close family friend, but suddenly, she became an enemy. To this day, I still have no idea what caused this change in mindset. I only know the devastation that it caused within my family.

This "leader" had an immense desire for power and would do whatever it took to ensure that she kept it. This involved a great deal of injustice, including numerous instances of shaming people publicly and embarrassing people for no reason. She handled conflict in the most hurtful and rude way possible, never attempting to reason or find solutions. Rather, she was bent only on strengthening the hold she had on others, even if it was at the expense of her former friends.

There were many times when she publicly shamed me in front of my peers. Considering what I was already going through, this had an extremely negative effect on me. I also began to notice how her actions affected my family. She attacked my father the most viciously, which led to his own depression. This, in turn, had a massive impact on our family's collective mood.

I grew angry and turned my sorrow into hate. I began to have violent dreams involving this particular person, and it started to consume me. I began to change the way I acted and responded to things, becoming short-tempered, angry, and violent. I would lash out unexpectedly at whoever was in my way.

It was strange; I only held disdain for this one person, yet I could never direct any of these feelings toward her. Instead, I lashed out at anyone else I could. These feelings were consuming my very being, and I needed help.

Forced To Get Help

I had **zero** intentions of seeing any psychiatrists. I was not crazy, and I didn't need some shrink asking me about my feelings. I tried to explain this to my parents, but it was no use. In reality, I *did* desperately need help. However, I couldn't accept help, because that would mean admitting that I had a problem.

I was terrified that they would discover that there was something *wrong* with me. I wasn't prepared to deal with any of the suggestions they would have for healing myself. I was *not* going to cry in front of anyone. I was *not* going to share my feelings, and I definitely was *not* going to let them label me as crazy. I felt completely fine, and I was convinced that I could deal with my own problems by myself. I didn't need help from someone who thought they knew me, just because they had a fancy degree that said so.

After countless heated arguments with my parents, I eventually had no choice. I had to see the psychiatrist. However, I made up my mind that I would remain silent, and waste both the psychiatrist's time and my parents' money to prove a point!

This tactic lasted for about two minutes, until I found out how cool and down-to-earth this shrink actually was. I had previously thought of psychiatrists as these wacky, apathetic weirdos, who wanted to show me ink blots and ask me how I felt about everything. That's why I was so surprised to find out that my psychiatrist was so incredibly normal. She was fairly young, probably mid-30s, and was quite pretty with her blonde hair pulled back into a loose ponytail. She didn't force anything, and she seemed genuinely interested in me and what I had to say. I had never experienced an adult, especially one in a position of relative authority, showing me so much respect. I was usually just treated like a little boy whose opinions meant nothing.

She got me talking without my realizing it, and once she slammed out her first cuss word, I *knew* I could trust her!

It was incredibly refreshing just to be able to talk with someone about everything I was experiencing, but also to be free to voice it in whatever manner I desired. I didn't have to be polite or hold anything back. I was allowed to just let go and get everything off my chest.

However, once I let it slip that I had been having

violent dreams and fantasies about another person's eventual death, and that I had been having suicidal thoughts, things changed. She did not act disgusted with me, as I had anticipated, but rather became even more concerned with my story. I could tell she had empathy and compassion for what I was going through. I can't even begin to explain how good it felt to me, to finally let loose, break my vow of silence, and not be rejected, but rather accepted! This was the first major turning point in my life, and without this experience, I honestly don't know where I would be today.

After the session, I was quickly referred and put on a mix of anxiety and depression medication. To be honest, I was so emotionally, physically, and spiritually drained at this point in my life, I welcomed it. I was so tired of the daily stomach pain that consumed my life that I was willing to try anything to stop it. In fact, I had grown so accustomed to the pain, I was actually shocked to find out that it might eventually go away with the right medication. I was still skeptical at first, because I didn't think the pain was being caused by my mind. I mean, it was real pain, right there in the pit of my gut. So how could my mind be the cause of that? But I figured if my mind was causing the pain, then my mind could stop the pain. If this medication could help my mind to do that, then more power to it!

Medication

Getting on medication was the best thing that ever could have happened to me. People often have very strict views about medication, more of which I will address in the final chapter, but the main problem I have with these people is that most of them have never experienced it for themselves.

They have never experienced what it is like to be truly hopeless—to hate themselves so much that they would rather die than continue living. They have never experienced the level of inner pain required to tempt them to take their own lives. They have never been stuck staring into space for days on end, nor felt like a load of bricks had just toppled upon them, virtually gluing them to their beds.

If you have never been the victim of depression, then you CANNOT comment on whether medication is morally or ethically wrong. Until you've been there and experienced the pain and the relief for yourself, you have no right to judge, call it a scam, or make any statements about whether it does or does not work.

I've been there, and I look at medication like this:

Let's say you're on a large ship that gets caught in a violent storm. The huge swells rock the boat, and the deck is pounded by mammoth waves. The crew is rushing feverishly to secure slack lines and do everything in their power to keep the boat afloat. Just then, a rogue wave hits the port side, and it knocks you off balance. You trip over the railing and plummet into the raging sea below. As you enter the cold, dark water, the storm seems to takes on a new intensity. The waves grow taller and crash down upon you with immense force. The constant blows take the breath from your lungs and thrust you deeper below the surface. You feel lost, and you're sure you're going to die.

Just then, a crew member on the boat yells from the side, "We're over here! Swim to us!"

This snaps you back into reality, but it's no use. What the crew can't realize is that you are out of breath, out of energy, and are unable to even see the boat or the safety that accompanies it.

However, just then, the boat's doctor throws a life preserver to you. You quickly reach out to grab it. It takes all your might to hold on, but it allows you to stay on the surface long enough to not only catch your breath, but also catch a glimpse of the boat.

You summon all of the energy left in you, and then in a flash, you make a mad dash toward the boat. It's not easy, as the waves continue to pound you from all sides. But equipped with the energy and perspective that the life preserver provided, you are able to reach the boat and finally get your feet back on solid ground!

I hope you can see the point I'm trying to make through this story. The storm represents the challenges or issues that we may face in life. Some, we may see coming, and others, we may not. But we all must deal with obstacles in life, whether we like it or not.

Through the whims of nature, some people will fall into the middle of the storm, and others may not. It does not make you "different" or "less" in some way if you happen to get knocked off your feet. It just means that you're human. Some of us, if we react quickly enough, may be able to grab hold and pull ourselves back onto the boat on our own. Or perhaps, if those around us take immediate action, they may be able to save us.

As for the rest, you are now trapped in a raging storm with no means of escape. Some will call to you, saying, "Just swim to us! We are right here!" Or in other words, "Be happy! Look at all the great things you have to live for!"

What these people don't realize is that you may not know how to swim. Perhaps you need help. Maybe you're so exhausted and out of breath that you have no energy left to make the journey back toward the boat.

Imagine if, just as the doctor was about to throw you the life preserver, the man yelling to you to "just swim" stopped the doctor and grabbed the preserver from him, claiming that it will do no good and you need to do this on your own.

This is the same as a licensed physician offering you a prescription for a medication that could save your life, and others telling you that you don't need it. It's easy for these people to say such things, as they have their feet firmly planted on the ground and are in no danger of drowning themselves. The physician knows what is best for you, and therefore his judgment is the only one that should be valid to you.

The life preserver represents medication, whether it be anti-depressants, anti-anxiety, or any other form of medication. Medication doesn't solve the root issue, which is that you're still in the middle of the ocean and need to get out. However, what it does provide is a means to get you to safety. It can allow you to catch your breath and give you the perspective you need in order to start moving toward safety.

If you're at the point where you have lost all hope and can no longer see the boat, then the only way to survive is with the assistance of a life preserver. Don't listen to those who are unable to give you an unbiased opinion. Only trust those who truly love you, and your licensed physician. If he says it would be wise for you to take some form of medication and writes you a prescription, you would be a fool not to take the life preserver. You would be choosing to battle the storm alone.

The route back to safety may not be the easiest. You may encounter rough seas and unforeseen obstacles in your path. But with the right perspective, determination, and support, it is more than possible to reach the boat and plant your feet on solid ground once again.

Another factor to take into consideration is the chemicals inside our bodies. Our physical minds and bodies are made up of many different chemicals in specific amounts. Eventually, some of these chemicals may become imbalanced for whatever reason, and this causes a physical reaction. You may become anxious, or you may start to feel low on energy. You may become aggressive, or you may feel depressed. This is a *physical* response to the chemical imbalances in your body. What the medications do is return the chemical levels in your system to a balanced state. Medications do not fix the problem that caused the imbalances in the first place, but they do put you back into a place where you are actually able to fix them for yourself.

This is why it's important to set yourself up with the proper support system to make sure you stick to the core issues and deal with them. There are so many variables to consider, and no two circumstances are the same. However, with the right support, I believe any situation can be brought under control, and in time return to a state of normalcy.

Note: Don't worry if you feel that I didn't explain the support system in detail. I will go into it in more depth in the final chapter.

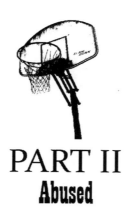

PART II
Abused

"Silence is what abusers love. Question them, confront them, report them. Never conform or surrender. The only way to ensure nothing changes is by doing nothing."

Home Sweet Home

In the summer of 2009, my family and I finally returned to our home in Canada. I thought–hoped–

that things would return to the way they had once been. I longed for a sense of normality. Instead, I now found myself with a bad case of culture shock, struggling to integrate back into a society that I used to feel was mine.

I quickly noticed that I was extremely awkward with people socially, and casual conversion became something that brought on considerable anxiety for me. Encounters that I used to take for granted became a huge burden for me, and I would often go out of my way to avoid them.

One example is buying groceries. I dreaded the casual "small talk" one normally partakes in with the cashiers when checking out of stores. Even these quick, relatively meaningless encounters became a source of high anxiety. I would think about the exchange long before it was going to take place, leading to sweaty armpits and a dry tongue. After a while, I began to avoid shopping alone all together. If I was with someone, then they could handle the social aspect for the both of us. But if I was alone, I would usually avoid the situation altogether.

Occasionally, I would come across a store with a

"self check-out service," in which case I would take full advantage. The blinking lights and pixilated screens seemed far less daunting than face-to-face interaction.

I had, in a sense, become unsociable. I was no longer striving toward acceptance, but rather avoiding it as a whole. I became a zombie in my own house, not fully dead, yet not fully alive. Something drastic had to be done. I did not want to live this way, and I was ready for whatever change that meant.

High School

In September of that same year, I made the decision to attend a high school. This was a big step for me, as I had previously been home-schooled for my entire life. I knew nothing of what the life of a "regular" student entailed, and I was petrified by the chasm of the unknown.

You may be thinking, *"You were home-schooled, so you must have been anti-social to start with!"*

This is a common misconception. Home-schooled kids are not always anti-social or children with special needs. My mother was actually a certified high school teacher, and she taught middle and high school kids when I was very young. She had all of the qualifications to provide my sister and me with a great education, and she did just that.

My mother was also unwaveringly passionate about spending time with her children. She didn't want to ship us off every day from nine until three, and then hear about what we did after the fact. She wanted to experience what we experienced by being a part of it. She took us on countless field trips to zoos, aquariums, science museums, you name it! It was not only fun and educational, but it was also an integral part of our development from children to teenagers.

During this time, she and my father were able to instill positive beliefs in us and encourage thinking outside the norm—not conforming to what society wanted us to believe, but rather using critical thinking skills to make our own decisions about what was right for us. Because of this, I had the strength to stand up to peer pressure and avoid doing many things that I would regret. I'm extremely thankful for what my parents did for me and for the education they gave me. I would have never become the man I am today without their care, dedication, and guidance. They truly are my best assets and my greatest inspiration, so thank you, Mom and Dad!

Eventually, however, the desire to play in coordinated high school sports became too great. I found myself longing to attend a high school to accommodate those desires. This also would provide a perfect opportunity to work through my social imbalances, which were causing so much strain on my daily life. So, in the summer of 2011, I attended my first *public* high school.

I had no idea of what to expect. My first experiences were incredibly awkward, and I really struggled to make friends. This was unfamiliar territory for me, as I grew up being extremely social and friendly. However, being absent from interaction with my peers for so many of my formative years left me at a huge social disadvantage. This led to a very difficult freshman year. On the bright side, though, I did discover my love for basketball, which turned out to become my major focus for the next four years of my life.

Basketball

I began to focus heavily on basketball, and I quickly became a pretty good player. I continued to practice incredibly hard over the summer until, when I returned for my sophomore year, I was the best player on my team. Not only that, but I actually ended up playing on the senior team—playing against juniors and seniors as a sophomore—and becoming one of the top scorers in my league. I finished the year strong and ended up taking home Second Team All-Star honors in my league.

I came to realize that my dream of playing at the next level was a definite possibility for me, but I knew that I would have to abandon my small school in order to have that opportunity. So, in the summer of 2011, I switched schools. In doing so, I opened myself up to new possibilities and experiences — both positive and negative.

A New School and a New Coach

My new school was much larger than the previous one. Though most of the culture shock had worn off, nothing could have prepared me for what I would experience in those next couple of years.

Before attending the school, I was warned that it would be tough. The basketball tradition there was far greater and the competition level much higher. I was specifically warned about the coach of the team, particularly that he was extremely intense and wasn't afraid to get in his players' faces.

In preparation for making my decision, I attended a few games to observe this coach in action and see if he was something I could handle. Though he was intense, I realized that this was exactly how most college and university coaches would treat their players. Therefore, I thought it would be a good way of preparing for the next level.

The first few months leading up to the season went great. This new coach and my new team really pushed me hard, and I grew as a player because of it. The trouble started when the season was about to begin. I noticed that my coach was becoming more and more intense as the season grew near, but I brushed it off, thinking it was normal.

However, things soon took a dramatic turn for the

worse. My coach began to verbally assault many of his players, myself included. He challenged us mentally, to the point of breaking.

I distinctly remember a particular conversation I had with a referee a few games into the season. The second half was about to begin, and I was waiting for the ref to hand me the ball so I could inbound it. Without provocation, the ref uncharacteristically turned to me and said, "So you're the new whipping boy, eh?"

I wasn't sure how to respond. I knew that I felt abused and belittled by this man, but I had thought that maybe it was all in my head. But when I realized that this referee, with whom I had previously had no contact, could see that I was the coach's "whipping boy" after only 20 minutes of play, then I knew that the problem was far more serious than I had imagined.

Being abused in practice was one thing. As many of the other players also experienced the same treatment, the abuse didn't affect us so much. It actually brought us closer together, as we could joke about it after practice and make light of the situation, although it affected many of us far more deeply than we would ever let on. What bothered me much more was when he would belittle us during games.

Now, I don't want you to think I'm some little sissy who can't take a competitive coach. On the contrary, I *love* competition and am actually quite intense myself. But when a coach starts screaming "YOU SON OF A B*TCH!" during play, in front of your peers, it gets to you.

This was actually a common occurrence. He would rant and rave throughout the entire game, often specifically directing the majority of his attention at me. During each game, he cussed at me personally three to five times, and at the team 10 to 15 times.. We were frequently called "Selfish little pukes," "Dumb *sses," and "Dumber than a sack of horse sh*t."

He would also try to prevent us from talking to our parents about his behavior. He would go so far as to take us into another room after practice and lay into us for 45 minutes, either to prevent us from speaking out or to punish us for doing so.

In one instance in particular, I remember the coach laid into one of the less talented, more socially awkward players on our team. He had found out the name of a Christian rock band that this boy listened to, and he spent the better part of 30 minutes tearing him apart for it. On top of feeling that this was completely uncalled for, I also enjoyed this particular group myself. Because the coach didn't know this, it wouldn't have been obvious to him that I had gone home and shared my feelings on the matter with my parents.

Others must have done the same, because the following morning, we found ourselves in serious trouble. It had gotten back to our coach that some of the parents were upset with him, and he was livid. He then went so far as to say we weren't to discuss anything that happened during practices with *anyone,* especially our parents. He said we were a team, and what happened within our team should stay within our team. This was a huge red flag for me, as I recognized this as a telltale sign of an abuser.

It wasn't entirely serious, however. Sometimes his ramblings were so absurd that they were borderline hysterical. On one occasion, he somehow managed to compare us to prostitutes due to a lack of effort during one of our 6 AM practices. He mentioned something about putting $1,000 in the corner of the gym and saying that the first person to get it would get to keep it.

He then made the connection that our interest in the prize meant that we would sell ourselves out for money, and that we were no better than prostitutes.

I couldn't help but smirk. These types of "creative" analogies happened frequently, but they never got to me. They were far too ridiculous and absurd for me to actually waste my time listening to. So I found myself learning to make it look as if I was paying attention, when in reality I was saving my brain space for things that actually *mattered* in life.

On the other hand, I don't wish to make light of his actions, as they affected me deeply. Especially after all of the mistreatment I had endured in Thailand, I was already primed to be vulnerable to abusive behavior. I soon began to withdraw my emotions again, as I had done in Thailand, which pushed me into another downward spiral.

The problem with being the victim of abuse—whether verbal, physical, or sexual—is that it can be really tough to talk about. You feel almost embarrassed about it, like it's somehow your fault. This couldn't be further from the truth, as it is in NO WAY anybody's fault if they are being abused... other than the abuser.

But that doesn't change how you feel, and if no one comes to your aid and steps up to say, "This is wrong," then it's easy to feel hopeless and alone.

My parents eventually caught on to my withdrawn behavior and quickly discovered the cause of the damage. Instinctively, they wanted to jump in and save me from my abuser, but I persuaded them not to. I kept telling them that they would only make it worse.

Since I had such a passion for basketball, I never even entertained the idea of quitting. So I felt trapped under this man's control and didn't want to do anything that would cause me more unwanted attention. Again, this is a classic sign of a victim of abuse, but of course I didn't see it that way.

No Help?

What really bothered me was that no one came to my aid.

Especially those in power. Many saw what was happening, saw how it was effecting me, but instead chose to turn a blind eye.

It was truly heartbreaking, because it was the very people that were put in these positions of power who were abusing it by letting abuse take place under their watch. Even while they knew without a doubt it was happening, they chose what was best for them rather than stepping in and making it stop.

Suicide Part II

I again felt hopeless, and with hopelessness comes a sense of desperation for change. Therein lies the problem: how can there be change without hope? If you felt there was a way in which you *could* change the situation, then there would be some hope. So, naturally you resort back to the only thing you ever have control over: your life.

This time, I struggled with suicidal thoughts much more intensely than I did in Thailand. This time was worse, because it was the second time in such a short period that the state of my life had reached this low point. I was afraid my whole life was going to be like this, and I didn't want any part of it.

I knew that my parents were worried about me,

but I didn't even care. Something that I normally would be sickened by—the thought of my parents fearing for my life—didn't even faze me. I again became numb to the world around me. I struggled to get through the years.

Eventually, my senior season ended, and a new sense of relief filled my soul. Instead of working on my troubles, and properly dealing with them, I instead chose to move past them. I chose to leave them behind as a gloomy blur in the rear window of my life, where they drifted farther and farther from sight and settled into the darkest places inside of me. I longed for them to stay hidden forever, never to resurface. This would eventually come back to bite me, ultimately changing the course of my life forever.

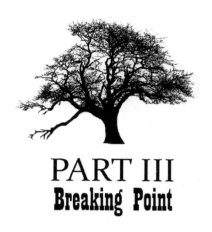

PART III
Breaking Point

"You will never know your breaking point until you reach it. Only then will you truly know your own limitations."

Goal Accomplished

However traumatic my high school may have been, it still served the original purpose that I intended it to: getting a scholarship to play at the next level. I wound up getting the opportunity to play for a team in the highest level Canada has to offer, the CIS. This is roughly the equivalent of division II basketball in the

US.

Still reeling from the difficulties faced during the last two years, I decided to move on and hope that time would heal my wounds.

Leaving Home

I didn't anticipate how hard moving out would be. I wasn't ignorant to the realities of living on my own, such as doing laundry, making food, tidying up after myself, commuting, buying essentials, etc. What I overlooked was the intense bond I shared with my family, and how much it would affect me once it was gone.

I had always loved my family, but after our struggles in Thailand, we definitely grew closer as a unit. We relied heavily on each other for guidance, sympathy, and encouragement. Once I realized I would be losing all these emotional comforts at once, I went into a state of panic. My family was my only constant throughout my life. They were my rock when I was scared, my guidance when I was lost, and my comfort when I needed to grieve. Even while my homes were constantly changing, along with my friends, schools, churches, and even countries, my family always remained. "Home" was no longer a *place* for me, but rather *people*—my people, my family. So by losing them, I felt I was losing a piece of myself that I had never been without before. I was completely petrified of how I would respond.

I had never thought much about how leaving home would affect me, largely because I thought it was something I simply had to do. It had been ingrained in me as a young boy that once you graduated high school, you would leave home and go to college. I further assumed that I would immediately find work after graduating, idealistically correlating a degree with some sort of monetary value.

I also thought I would find the girl of my dreams in college, we would date, and then we would live happily ever after! This simply isn't realistic, but by the time I figured that out, it was already too late. I was left completely unarmed in the battle of *real life*.

Rookie Hazing

Life did not get any easier once I was left to my own devices. My parents were gone, and I had to face university on my own.

I had to report to school for pre-season training two weeks before classes officially began. I was very afraid and extremely anxious.. I didn't know anybody on the team, nor could I anticipate what to expect. I basically had three major obstacles to face at once: playing on a new team at a much higher level of basketball, leaving my home and my family, and facing university and all the academic stresses that accompany it.

The physical side to training was incredibly demanding. We were doing two practices a day before the school year officially started. This usually meant two to three hours of hard basketball training, followed by some sort of cardio/agility training later in the day. That was tough, and I struggled to keep up. I had suffered an injury in the weeks leading up to this, and my poor cardio condition definitely showed as well.

As hard as it was physically, it was just as challenging mentally, as all of this stress on my body coupled with the stress on my mind. I was always anxious, and the same stomach issues I had faced in Thailand came back to plague me once again. I constantly thought I was going to be sick, which made all the physical work my body had to do nearly impossible.

I somehow managed to survive those first few weeks, and I finally got a couple of days off during the university's orientation. I thought I would use this time to take a step back and relax, letting my body and mind take a break and heal as best they could. My teammates, however, had different plans.

For whatever reason, "rookie hazing" has become commonplace in our modern society, especially for sports teams. I don't care what reasons people give for its prevalence, like "*It builds team chemistry*" or "*They need to be put in their place before [whatever].*" This is not the case. These excuses are just poorly veiled attempts to hide the real issue at hand: a cycle of abuse.

It's the same reason that abusive behavior often continues through multiple generations in families.

You would think that a boy who was abused as a child would be far more likely to avoid abusing his own child, especially since he knows the physical and emotional damage it causes. But in fact, victims of abuse are actually MORE likely to become abusive. First of all, this is how they were taught to behave. The idea that abuse is acceptable is ingrained during childhood, and that stays with many victims throughout their lives. There is also a certain level of shame, embarrassment, and guilt that follows these victims around. Instead of dealing with their emotions properly, through counseling and healing, they instead become abusers themselves to take back the power that was taken from them.

In the case of my team, the upperclassmen had scheduled a "rookie party" for that weekend, and it was mandatory. Basically, it was an excuse for them to do stupid things to us, in order to inflict the same level of embarrassment that had been inflicted upon them.

The main problem I had was that one of the things they often made rookies do was drink a ridiculous amount of liquor, often until they puked. This posed two serious threats for me. The first was my intense aversion to throwing up, and the second was that I don't drink. I've seen firsthand how alcohol can break apart families and destroy lives. I don't have a problem with others drinking around me, but I personally refuse to ever consume a drop of alcohol myself.

This got back to my teammates, and they weren't buying it. They also had no idea how strong my will was, so they thought they could easily persuade or force me into submission.

When it was clearly evident that they could not, they switched tactics and made me drink milk instead. This was a problem for me because milk is extremely hard to hold down in large quantities, and I was still terrified of puking. A huge part of me did not want to show up to the party, but I knew that if I had any hope of surviving on this team, I had to. So I did.

First, they made us strip down basically to our underwear, and they took humiliating pictures of us. Then we had our first "contest." We had to chug a can of beer and a shot, and then sprint around the block in our underwear for all to see. Obviously, I wasn't going to drink the liquor, so they instead poured two glasses of milk for me, filled to the brim.

This gave me a huge disadvantage, as milk is far

thicker and harder to consume, and I was given much more to drink than the others. My teammates said this was my fault for choosing not to drink alcohol (which actually would have been illegal, since I was underage).

The loser of this race would be punished by having to do a 30-second keg stand following the race. For those who don't know, a keg stand is when a participant does a handstand on top of a keg of beer, while others hold his legs up. Another person will hold the keg tap, attached to the keg with a short length of tubing, in the participant's mouth. In this disorienting and nauseating position, the participant tries to drink as long as possible.

I had no intention of doing this, so I really couldn't have cared less if I won or lost their little race. Nevertheless, when they said, "Go," we were off.

I drank the milk as fast as I could without making myself totally sick, trying my best to "accidentally" spill as much of the thick white substance as I could without getting caught. As I finished my first glass, others were finishing their shots and starting off around the block. I tried to increase my speed, but it was no use. I was well behind the pack and had no chance of catching up. I did my best to stay as close as possible, but I also didn't overdo it, as I knew I had no chance of escaping last place.

When I arrived back at the party, I was quickly swarmed by the others, already taunting me about my impending doom. I made it clear that I was still not going to drink, and that this wasn't going to change under any circumstances. They continued to harass me, but I stood my ground. I knew my limits, and I would not exceed them at the whim of some maniacs. I had no fear of getting punched or beaten, so physical intimidation wouldn't work on me. Eventually, they realized that I was not going to budge and finally moved on.

The next challenge involved doing wall sits. Another rookie and I were forced to sit against the jagged wall with our bare backs exposed. The sharp pain was the least of my worries, as they placed a broom handle on our legs and explained that if we let it drop, we would have to start over. They handed us our drinks—for me this meant more milk—and said that we had to consume the liquid and stay squatting for two minutes. This was especially difficult, because my legs were already shaking with fear and adrenaline, and the broom handle made it impossible to adjust my position even the slightest bit.

Near the end of the two minutes, it became almost too much to bear. I started grunting to fight the pain. This unleashed a torrent of insults that rained down upon me as I sat there, defenseless. I am not sure if it was the fire smoldering in my thighs or the rage in my heart, but I quickly shot back at them with insults of my own, calling into question their character, morals, and life values. Surprisingly, this had a serious impact on them, and I knew I had struck a sensitive spot.

They told me that I had just dug myself into a larger hole, but at this point I had already made up my mind that I would rather quit this team than comply with these morons any longer. The two minutes was up, and my fellow rookie and I collapsed to the ground. Our backs were torn up by the wall, but we hadn't the strength to stand and relieve our own suffering.

Not long after, the girls' basketball team arrived at the party with their own rookies that they were hazing. This led to many awkward forced interactions between some of the male and female rookies, and I knew I had seen enough.

I am a firm Christian and had zero desire to do anything that would shame myself, my family, or my God. What they were making these rookies do would surely accomplish that, and therefore I knew I must leave.

It was going to be a tricky procedure, but I knew it had to be done. My heart raced as I anticipated the repercussions of getting caught, but I chose to shove them to the back of my mind. I managed to eventually slip away from main action and began scouting out the front door. Though no one was near it, it was in plain view of most of the party and all those on the terrace outside.

I mustered up all of the courage I could, quickly grabbed my clothes, and eased my way through the door. Once through, I bolted around the corner and into the nearest bush. I was finally free, and I quickly clothed myself and set off toward campus.

You may be wondering why I was so nervous about being caught but not about them finding out later that I had left. Well, I was definitely concerned about this, but I also counted on the lack of clarity that usually accompanies a night of heavy drinking. In other words,

I figured they would be too drunk to even notice or remember that I had left. It ended up being the former.

Even though I fought through the entire episode and even left early, it still affected me greatly. Though I may have made light of a few situations, there was far more to it. Ultimately, it was an extremely traumatic experience for me. The fear and terror I felt during that night triggered some of my old issues from back in Thailand and from my high school coach. This left me in an extremely vulnerable state, as I was now anxious and scared basically all of the time.

This constant state of anxiety and fear took its toll on me, and I once again began to lose any sense of joy in life.

Alone

Another area that was extremely problematic for me was that I didn't have any sort of support system in place to help me up when I started into my downward spiral again.

I still remember my first sleepless night away from

my family. I spent the night wedged into the corner where my bed met the wall, hoping and praying for some sort of peace—a release from this constant and unrelenting fear.

Most nights were like this. I was overwhelmed by fear, which led to panic, which led to sorrow, weeping, reflecting, and finally... *nothing*. That was the worst. The absence of any feelings was my only means of protection. Since I couldn't control which feelings I had, I instead learned to turn them off and feel nothing. Eventually, this led to severe depression, as I became even more withdrawn and unable to take pleasure in anything.

I was completely alone, and I had no motivation or energy to go out and socialize with those around me. In addition, basically all of the kids around me were getting drunk and having sex, which is totally out of alignment with who I am. I longed for interaction with others, but I was incapable of making it happen by myself.

My only sense of relief would come when my parents would visit me for a weekend, or when I got the chance to Skype with them over the internet. But the goodbyes quickly became heavier than the joys that came from spending a couple of days together, so I eventually started encouraging them to stay away.

I began to dread the days again, and I became clinically depressed for a third time. There was no thought of suicide this time. It was more just a sense of complete emptiness. I turned off my senses and lived without trying to feel anything for weeks. I was constantly tired, and I started taking frequent naps, which I hadn't done since I was five years old.

The days blurred together, and my grades plummeted. I no longer saw the point in anything anymore. I also didn't have energy to do anything, even to think. I just turned off my brain and coasted through my day.

I began contemplating purposely playing poorly in practice so that I would not be chosen to go on the trips for out-of-town games. We had to fly all over Canada, and it became a burden for me. Ironically, the less I cared about my basketball performance, the better I would play. I became fearless and started making huge improvements, and I would sink a number of very difficult shots at every practice. I was even the best shooter on my team for a stretch of over a month and started to get playing time in games because of it. This should have been great news, but again, I didn't care. My life was basically over in my mind, and all I was trying to do was finish off the year so that I could hopefully move on to something—anything—better.

Christmas Break

I started reaching my breaking point just before Christmas break. I began to lash out at teammates (some of whom deserved it), which was very uncharacteristic of me. I also began swearing in practices much more frequently and started to become a disturbance for the coach. I still remember the look of bewilderment on his face when I drop-kicked a ball into the rafters after losing a meaningless pick-up game. This could normally warrant being kicked out of practice, but since it was so out of character for me, he didn't know how to respond. Honestly, I didn't know how to respond, either.

I had become something I didn't want to be: someone who was angry and bitter. Someone who took joy in nothing and lived in constant fear. Christmas break finally arrived, and I set off for home without any expectations about how the visit would go.

The Decision

My parents knew I was in a dismal state, and they confronted me about it as soon as I got home. They kept reminding me that I could always leave university and return home if I deemed it necessary. This always frustrated me, as I kept telling them it wasn't that simple. I couldn't even consider coming home, because it would mean quitting.

I know it sounds cliché, but I seldom quit anything in my life, and doing so is extremely hard for me. This was also the dream I had worked so hard for during the previous four years, so of course I couldn't even imagine giving it up. The problem was I didn't even enjoy this dream that I had accomplished, but I still couldn't find it in myself to quit.

My intention was always to return to university and finish off the year as best I could, and then decide where to go from there. My parents weren't entirely sure that this was the best idea. They were very nervous that things would not improve, but rather worsen over the final semester—so much so that they were worried about my personal safety.

My mother even told me recently that there had been times when she didn't want to hang up the phone with me. She was so worried about my state of mind that she was terrified I was on the verge of self-harm.

On top of that, I also began to experience extreme stomach discomfort over the break again, just like I had in Thailand. I was terrified that this would be the straw that broke the camel's back. I could barely handle myself as it was, even without stomach problems. How could I cope with this additional burden?

I began to wrestle with the idea of returning home. Each time, I would quickly cast it aside. What was more important to me: finishing my year of university just for the sake of finishing, or coming home and getting the serious help that I needed? The choice was brutally difficult to make, and either decision was going to be incredibly difficult to carry out.

I still remember crying into a pillow just after midnight with my mother sitting next to me, telling me

I had to make a decision. My father was going to take me back to my dorm the following morning, and either he was dropping me off, or we were getting my things.

It was the toughest decision I have ever been faced with, and I begged my mother to make it for me. She refused, as this was my life and I was the one who had to live with the consequences of my actions.

Clutching a pillow with all my might, body tense and rigid, I finally mustered up the courage to say, "I'm going to stay home and get help."

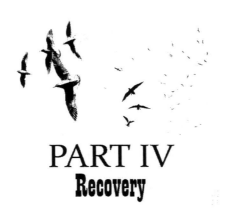

PART IV
Recovery

"Sometimes it takes more strength to allow yourself to be weak than to pretend that you are strong."

Long Road Ahead

Now that the decision was finally made, it was time to start the real work. My father and I departed first thing in the morning. It was four hours each way, and we drove mostly in silence. I was afraid of what was to come.

When we arrived, I had to complete the shameful task of informing my coach and my teammates that I wouldn't be finishing the season with them. Then, I had to sneak all my belongings out of my dorm room and into the car, not wanting to be seen in my humiliation. Finally, I had to talk to the dorm management, tell them my situation, and give them my keys.

No one saw this coming, and everyone was completely shocked. I did my best to explain that this wasn't anybody's doing and that no one could have seen this coming because I was great at hiding my emotions. Both of those statements were complete lies.

How could I bluntly tell someone that they were indeed one of the main reasons for this decision; that their childish, immature hazing rituals sent me over the edge; and that if anyone had taken the time to look past themselves and see that I needed help, maybe this all could have been avoided?

Saying any of that wouldn't have changed the past. Therefore, I decided to keep it hidden. I let them think that they had nothing to do with it, since that's what they ultimately wanted to hear.

I faced a long journey ahead. I didn't want these

Safe Place

This was the first step in my healing process. I needed to find a safe place to finally relax and let go of my anxiety. For me, this meant coming home. More specifically, this meant being with my family. You wouldn't believe how extraordinary it feels to finally be able to breathe peacefully after months of living in constant fear. Feeling *nothing* was the greatest feeling on earth.

I believe that a good friend of mine, who has had similar mental health struggles, put it wonderfully with this quote:

"You never know happy unless you've known sad. You never take for granted the

days when you feel average because those ones are spectacular. An average day is a great day."

It was truly incredible to feel safe again, and this was something that I definitely used to take for granted. Before I left for university, I couldn't wait to leave the house. At that time, I was becoming easily agitated by those I had spent the prior 19 years of my life with, and I thought it was their fault. I figured that I needed to leave, or else I would go insane. However, it seems as if going insane was an inevitable outcome that I had no chance of avoiding.

Being humbled in the way that I was—basically running back into my parents' arms and saying that I had made a mistake—truly was the best thing that ever could have happened to me. I was not wrong for leaving home, and it wasn't something I wouldn't normally be prepared for. If my mental health had been as it should be, none of the challenges at university would have been a major problem for me. Instead, however, I chose to believe the lies I had fed to myself: that I didn't need to deal with my problems, that I was fine the way I was.

This ultimately led to complete self-destruction. If I had dealt with my problems earlier, when I should have, then none of my issues would have resurfaced with the vengeance that they did.

Nevertheless, I was now living in the reality that I had created for myself. I wasn't about to sulk in the "what ifs." I was focused on my future and resolved not to let my past influence my future anymore.

Counseling

I decided that the next step in my long-term recovery was to talk about my problems. This ended up being much harder than I ever could have imagined.

I was ahead of most patients, however, in the sense that I had chosen to be there on my own terms. Most clients that counselors see are forced to be there and are solely bent on staying silent. I, on the other hand, at least had the internal desire to find healing and hope—even if it meant rehashing events that I had tried so hard to forget.

I struggled to bring up events that I didn't want to

admit took place, starting with Thailand and eventually leading to my coach and my university. It astounded me how little I could remember at first—how my brain had hidden my pain for my own good. But as soon as I started with one story, another would then come to mind. I would find myself getting very worked up as I relived these unjust events.

Even though I knew most of what the counselor would say, it still helped to hear it from someone else, especially someone of high stature. Sometimes, even though we *know* something, we may not *believe* it due to doubt in ourselves. But once we hear it from someone else who has no ulterior motive, it becomes more real to us.

My counselor also allowed me to slow things down and not rush my healing process. Since I was home now, I felt immense pressure to figure myself out as quickly as I could and start pulling my own weight. I felt guilty and embarrassed. I wanted to get back to "normal" as quickly as I could. Luckily, my counselor did a fantastic job of explaining the process to me. Healing can't really be measured by "fast" and "slow." It's an eternal process, and only I could know how long it would take. The only thing she could guarantee was that it wouldn't happen overnight, and she said I should let go of the stress of trying to make it happen.

Medication

You already know my philosophy in regards to starting medication: if you need it, don't hesitate to take it. It won't solve your problems, but it will put you in a place where you can solve your problems.

In my case, I was experiencing a severe case of both anxiety and depression. Mundane events would cause me panic, so much so that I would often avoid them. This meant that I basically couldn't leave the house. I was scared to go to my local gym, for fear of seeing people who expected me to be at university. I couldn't hang out with old friends. I couldn't play pickup basketball, and I especially couldn't hang out with girls. It sounds kind of funny, but it was very serious, and I needed help with it.

It got so bad that I started having panic attacks in my counseling sessions—the very things that were the most beneficial in my healing process. In addition, my sleeping patterns were a mess. I was tired all the time, but I couldn't fall asleep until very late. Then I would find myself sleeping for more than 10 hours, only to wake up still very tired. This cycle didn't allow me to live very productive days, and it was horrible for the tasks I was attempting to accomplish. I needed help for both my anxiety and my depression, and my counselor agreed.

Once I began taking anti-depression/anti-anxiety pills, things got better. The change was not immediate, as it takes a while for medication to start kicking in. But once the pills did start taking effect, I noticed an extreme difference in the way that I saw the world. I wasn't the only one, either. My parents, closest family, and friends also noticed big differences in my day-to-day life. These pills were not a permanent solution, but they allowed me to face my fears and deal with the issues that I needed to, in order to become healthy once again.

Spiritual

As I mentioned before, I'm a Christian. I won't try to push my faith on you, but it is an important part of my story, as my spiritual life played a huge role in my complete healing.

I would never consider my spiritual life as being perfect. In fact, it's probably never even been good. I've always been a good person, someone who truly cares for his neighbor and wants to see them happy. I didn't do drugs or sleep around, or really do anything that was considered "taboo" by the church. I thought that this made me a good Christian and that God and I were great friends. However, I soon saw how one-sided our relationship really was.

I personally believe that you can never truly experience God until you have put him above everything else you have. This can be extremely hard to do, especially in our North American society. We can basically get whatever we want, whenever we want, so why would any of us "need" God?

I sure didn't. I loved him and wanted to be great friends with him—just not enough to actually turn off my computer or the TV.

This had all came crashing down in an instant when I found myself curled up in a ball at two in the morning repeating to myself, "Jesus, I need you. Jesus,

I need you..."

This had happened less than two weeks into my university adventure. I was terrified and alone. I didn't know what to do to make the pain inside stop. The terror and sorrow were too much to bear, and I honestly did not know what to do. So I went to the only one, the only thing, that I had: "Jesus, I need you."

I must have repeated the phrase a million times over the few weeks that followed, as it gave me comfort. I began literally walking with God, as I would often go exploring nature around me, talking to him as I went.

At that point, I couldn't have cared less if God wasn't even real. Just believing in him encouraged me and gave me hope. I also found that talking to him about my situations really helped me feel better. I didn't do any fancy prayer. I didn't fall to my knees or speak in some Biblical language. I simply talked to him like I would a friend, and therefore he became one.

Eventually, my doubts about him were completely put aside as I began to truly experience him fully: his goodness, his mercy, and especially, his love!

Even though my trip to university was by far the

hardest thing I have ever had to go through–considering all that had led up to that point–if I had to do it all over again, I would do the same thing. I have become a changed person because of it. What my friend said is true: you really can't experience happiness, TRUE happiness, without first experiencing sadness. You can only be as high as you have been low... and boy have I experienced low. I've found new meaning in life, and it has allowed me to experience the wonders of each and every day just that much better.

72

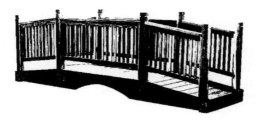

PART V
Advice For Others

"Asking for help is not weakness, but rather, pretending you are strong enough on your own is."

Find Strength in the Struggle

Here's the thing. First and foremost, I want to let you know that I have been there. I am not someone who claims to be a professional in human psychology, but I have been there myself. Truthfully, I will probably be there again. My counselor told me that anxiety and depression will probably be things I will suffer with for the rest of my life, because I am already susceptible to them both due to my past. This was kind of a heavy blow for me, since my whole purpose in coming home was to get better and become fully healed so that I wouldn't have to deal with these struggles ever again. When I mentioned this to her, she said that just because I may struggle with it, doesn't mean that it will ever affect me in the same way that it used to. Because I have dealt with these issues so many times in the past, I now know how to properly handle them in the future. This means I am actually more prepared than the average person to deal with anxiety and depression. I am now able to better recognize the early warning signs and address them before they become a problem. So please, if you are someone who deals with anxiety and depression and are looking for an answer, take what I say seriously. I am not trying to sell you anything and have no ulterior motives, other than to make sure YOU know that this will pass... and that YOU will become a stronger person because of it.

In addition, if you are not someone who is currently struggling with the above mentioned disorders, then please don't feel as though these principles don't apply to you. I believe we all suffer from different forms of depression/sadness in our lives at one time or another—though with varying degrees of intensity. This advice should be heard by all, since it is practical, beneficial, and easily understood. It can't hurt to be aware of these things if they ever should arise in your future, or even the future of someone you care about. So please, truly take in what I have to say with an open mind, and hopefully I will be able to add a little hope into your life.

Try to notice the signs as early as possible!

Just like with anything, the earlier you catch it, the less damage it can do. This can be especially difficult if it is your first time struggling with depression, since you don't necessarily know what signs to look for. But as you walk through your life's journey, with time you will better understand what makes you tick, thereby allowing yourself to notice when things are starting to get "out of whack."

I understand that if you are *already* suffering from depression, then this tip may not help you. However, if you are like me, then depression may be something you will be more susceptible to in your life. Therefore, it is worth understanding how and when it affects you the most. This is not a death sentence in the least, but I realize it is not something you necessarily want to hear. The last thing I wanted to hear was that this was something I would have to struggle with for my entire life. BUT keep in mind that just because we are more vulnerable, does NOT mean we will live a life full of sorrow and emptiness. We are actually the lucky ones because we will be able to experience joy in areas that most people take for granted. You can't experience true happiness without first experiencing sadness. Therefore, just imagine how happy we are now capable of being, considering what we have gone through! And if we take the time to learn how to deal with our issues—as you are doing right now!-then we can be prepared for whatever life throws at us. We can actually deal with life's challenges better than those who aren't as strong as we are.

That being said, here are some signs to look for that you may be on the verge of depression and may need to consider getting help:

Loneliness

This is a HUGE trigger for me. I am someone who needs the company of others to fuel my passions and desires for life. I never feel quite as energized as I do after spending quality time with those I love. That's why it was so incredibly important for me to find friends quickly when I was in university. My main problem was that I didn't have the chance to find these friends right away, as I was required to report two weeks before school actually started. This only left my teammates, and though some of them were incredible people whom I still love today, a few of them were extremely negative and sent me into a downward spiral before I even had the chance to create a safety net for myself.

Once other students did arrive on campus, I no longer had the desire to go out of my way to meet them. By not seeking out other friends, I set myself up for massive failure in the future.

Loneliness is very likely to be a trigger, to some extent, for us all. We are all human, and thus have an innate desire to "want" and feel "wanted." It is what makes us special, and what makes life such an incredible privilege to live! However, this is a double-edged sword, and we must be careful to understand both sides of the equation.

Bottom line: Don't allow yourself to become completely isolated from the world. Do not put yourself in positions where you have to rely on yourself to go out and seek the attention of others. If this means *not* leaving your family/friends for a while, so be it. It is never easy to leave your family, friends, and other loved ones behind; that can be an especially difficult experience for anyone. If leaving is something you feel you must do, then just make sure you are already in a *good* place mentally to begin with–something I was not–while also making sure you have a support system set up to help you succeed. This could mean making sure you have some friends where you are going, keeping in regular contact with those you have left behind, or even setting up appointments with a counselor once in a while, just to talk and keep a regular connection with someone.

Seeing a counselor should not be seen as a sign of weakness, and you don't have to be in a state of full-blown depression to take the leap and see one. Catch yourself before you fall, and just have regular visits to keep everything in order, even if it's just once a month. Trust me, it can save you A LOT of trouble in the future.

A major tragic event/A series of difficult events

Life happens, and it isn't always pleasant. People die, relationships end, and tragedy strikes. I don't mean to make light of these horrible occurrences. I just want to get the point across that they DO happen, and happen to us all. Death is a great example. You never plan it. You never look forward to it. But you have no way of stopping it. It is something we all have to deal with, whether we're young or old. Since preventing it is out of the question, we can only prepare ourselves to deal with it in the best way that we possibly can.

So far, there have been three major deaths that have affected me personally. Two great friends of mine were taken long before their time in separate, tragic events, and my grandpa passed away.

Though it was extremely hard to see my grandpa go, it wasn't unexpected. He had been fighting with diabetes for most of his life and had actually fought a few years longer than we thought he would. I do miss him greatly, and I'm saddened by his death. I was well prepared for it to happen though, and was therefore able to deal with it even before it took place.

This wasn't the case with my other friends. The first one was a young girl that I grew up with. She was actually my sister's friend, but she was extremely kind and went out of her way to befriend me also. Her death happened so suddenly and so unexpectedly that I didn't know what to do.

I still remember sitting in my final block of the day at school–woodworking–and glancing down at my phone. I saw two missed calls and three new messages. I knew that this wasn't good. I quickly hid myself in the corner to see what had happened and found out that my dear friend had passed away from a disease she'd acquired on the missionary trip she was on. It was so unexpected that her parents didn't even have a chance to reach her before she had passed.

This was incredibly hard to me to come to terms with, as it was my first major taste of what death does to those left behind. I did not process the situation well, and never properly allowed myself to grieve. This was a BIG mistake! Never try to make light of death. Even if it is someone who you may not think you even knew that well. It is human nature to feel sad and want to grieve for a loss, even if your grief is for those who will be more affected by it than yourself. Because of my poor processing, I am still struggling with her death to this day. It still doesn't seem real to me, and I fear it never will. I made a vow that I would never try to be overly strong during the passing of someone close to me. I swore that I would allow myself the time to grieve properly.

Therefore, when I found out that a great friend of mine from Thailand had passed in a freak car accident, I was strong enough to allow myself to be "weak." This can be especially hard for men in particular, but it is so important for the grieving process. I let the tears flow and gave my mind time to think and process.

If someone you love dies, don't feel as if you need to be "back to normal" quickly. It's OK to be sad and let yourself overcome the tragedy. Due to my experience with the first death, I was able to handle this one much better. Though I am still extremely distraught about the loss, I am OK with it and know that God has a bigger plan than I could ever understand. His perspective is much greater than my own, and I have to trust that he knows what he is doing. When I am able to do that, life becomes much simpler.

This doesn't only apply to death. Learning to grieve and allowing yourself to see the "big picture" is extremely beneficial for a multitude of challenges in life. This ability is invaluable and something that must be learned if not already acquired.

If you feel as though life just keeps throwing one unfair event after another, just hold on. I understand this better than most, and it sucks. There is nothing I can really say that can make it better. Just understand that life is like a roller coaster, with high points and low points. The key is to keep in mind the fact that low points are only temporary, and life will go on.

This doesn't mean that it doesn't hurt, and at times it may seem like it is too much to handle. But you can handle it! The cliché that life only gives you as much as *you* can handle isn't true. That is, if you are talking about handling everything alone. However, I DO believe that we can get through ANYTHING together, with the help and support of those around us. For you, his could be your family, your friends, your wife or husband, or even a counselor. Don't think you're so strong that you don't need others, and don't think you're so alone that others don't need you. We all need help, and the sooner we allow ourselves to *be* helped, the better off we will be.

Bottom line: Allow yourself to grieve. Gain perspective. Everyone faces trauma at some point, not just you. Learn to rely on others for support. Don't be afraid of getting help.

Major changes

This could mean moving, leaving for university, switching schools, or any other big change.

Change is never easy. It's something most of us dread; some more than others. I, for one, have always hated change and don't like being surprised. I enjoy knowing well in advance what is going to take place, so I can prepare myself mentally and emotionally. That isn't always going to happen. Life will throw you curve balls. It's not about avoiding them, it's about learning to catch them when they come, and realizing that sometimes you are going to get hit.

When we get hit or have a setback, we have to realize that it's how we *respond* to that setback that will determine how hard the impact will be. Those caught off guard are usually hit the hardest. Those who think that they are immune to life's challenges and obstacles will often be the most greatly affected when they come. If we instead prepare ourselves ahead of time, knowing that things may happen that we have no way of anticipating, then we can't be hit off guard.

That isn't to say that change isn't still hard to deal with. Two of the most challenging events in my life were moving to Thailand, and leaving for university. They challenged me in ways I never thought possible, allowing me to truly *find* myself and become stronger because of them.

Bottom line: Change is a part of life. It isn't easy or pleasant. However, the sooner we realize this, the easier these challenges will become. Don't allow yourself to stay ignorant of life's challenges, or you may find yourself blindsided by a pitch that you never saw coming!

Abusive situations

This is a subject extremely close to my heart. If you have been abused, bullied, or victimized in any way, then I am truly sorry. I personally would like to kick the crap out of ANYONE who attempts to hurt another human being. I hate bullies and abusers with a passion. However, we have to realize that they are often victims themselves. This is not always the case, as this world does have some evil people in it. But most of the time, people feel the need to abuse others in order to regain something they have lost through abuse.

This by no means is my way of saying that you shouldn't defend yourself. If someone is physically abusing you for whatever reason, and you think the only answer is to physically put a stop to it yourself, then by all means go for it. But I would strongly urge you to think hard on the matter and realize that a lot of the time violence only makes the situation worse for you.

I am neither promoting nor discouraging violence, but instead trying to help you judge what is the best course of action for your situation.

I wish I could give an easy, foolproof method to stop the abuse and obtain justice, but that isn't a realistic goal. Life is full of bullies, and it's up to those with honor and strength to stand up to them.

I would advise you to do *something,* however. In my own personal experience, bullies don't stop until confronted, either by you, your friends, your parents, teachers, those in authority, or even the police. Never be afraid to get help, no matter how much you are threatened. If the situation demands it, don't hesitate to seek police protection.

It won't be fun to make it stop. The process of freeing yourself from being victimized is not always pleasant. For me personally, it was one of the hardest things to do to leave my university, and the whole process was horrible. But once the dust had settled, I was extremely thankful for my decision, as I was now able to move on with my life freely.

Bottom line: I know being the victim sucks. There are few things worse. I wish I could tell you that everything is going to be all right, and I would love to personally beat the stuffing out of those who are hurting you. But that isn't realistic.

The key is to intelligently weigh the situation in your head, assessing the pros and cons of how to proceed, and then TAKE ACTION! Don't allow abuse to thrive. Stomp it out right away, and get those with power and authority on your side.

You can do it! You are brave and have immense courage within you. I know it's there. Now it's time to show the world!

Find a "Safe Place"

The key to my healing was to find a "safe place," a place where I could relax, have no distractions, and finally address my issues. For me, this meant coming home.

This isn't *always* possible–it wasn't when I was in Thailand–but whenever it is possible, I believe it definitely should be done.

A safe place for you may not be your home. It may mean a certain country or state, a friend's house, getting away for a bit on your own... only you know. But I would strongly encourage you to pursue this option, as it can be instrumental in getting your life back where you want it.

Force Yourself to Talk About It

This can be one of the hardest things you ever do in your lifetime... it was for me. Whether you feel embarrassed, ashamed, or even if it's just too painful to relive, it's worth working through it with a licensed professional, or at the very least with trusted loved ones.

You are not showing "weakness" by making the decision to see a counselor, but in fact, an immense amount of strength!

The first time I saw one, I had ZERO intention of saying anything or opening up. I was forced to go by my parents, and I was furious because of it. In the end, it turned out to be the greatest thing that could have happened to me at the time, and it allowed me to get my life moving in the right direction.

I should have seen another counselor while I was going through the abuse in high school, but I was too proud, or too ashamed to do so. This proved to be detrimental to my health, as these emotions brewed inside of me until I couldn't take it anymore and had to stop everything I was doing at the time to come home and get my life together.

That incident led to the second time I saw a counselor, completely by my own will this time. I still remember walking into her office and saying, "I have some major issues, I don't want to work on them, but I HATE where I am at right now and I know I need to. So let's get it done."

I ended up making one of the quickest and most radical transformations she had ever witnessed. She was amazed by my progress, but I honestly couldn't have done it without her. The reason I was so successful so quickly had much to do with two things. First, I am an EXTREMELY motivated person, so when I set my mind to something, it gets accomplished. Second, I did just that. I made up my mind that I was going to deal with my problems—not just talk about them—and finally be able to carry on with living my life to the fullest.

It is absolutely necessary to FULLY commit to the

process of healing if you want to get the most out of it. I'm not saying that recovery isn't possible if you don't, but it may take much longer and the results may not be as dramatic as you had hoped. Commit yourself to getting the healing you need, even if it means putting yourself out there in uncomfortable places and sharing parts of yourself in the safety of the counselor's office that you have kept hidden all your life. If you do this, then I have no doubt that you will once again be happy... and even better, you will thrive!

Seek Medication

I have harped on this a lot already, so you should already know my stance. To sum it up quickly, medication is a tool to help you get to where you are going. It will not "fix" you, but it can allow you to get to the point where you can then fix yourself.

My counselor actually gave me a great analogy that she uses when clients are resistant to the idea of medication. She said to imagine you broke your leg. Now, you wouldn't just stand up and say, "I can fix this myself." No, you would go to the hospital, get x-rays, set the bones, get a cast, allow the bones to heal, and then finally go to physiotherapy to strengthen the leg.

Medication is just one of those steps in the process of healing. Your broken heart shouldn't be treated any differently than a broken limb. There are real-life steps to be taken with a broken heart in order to properly heal it, and most people overlook them. As with a broken leg, when your heart is broken, the actual healing process might be too difficult and painful to complete on your own. Medication can ease the pain enough to allow you to get through it and truly heal.

Accept That You *May* Not "Know It All"

I'm going to be real with you.

You don't have all the answers.

And what's more, it's OK that you don't know have all the answers. We are only humans, small humans, living in an unimaginably massive universe. It is perfectly fine to not understand the internal matrix of the whole system, especially when you are young.

"The more I <u>know</u>, the more I realize I <u>don't</u> know." — Unknown

This is one of my favorite quotes, mainly because I feel that I can easily relate to it.

When I was really young, I didn't really know about anything. Once I grew, and my knowledge of my surroundings expanded, I began to gain the perception that I *knew everything*. No one could tell me anything, and I had opinions on just about any topic that you could bring up. This was a problem for two main reasons:

1. People *hate* being around "know it alls"

2. I actually didn't know everything... though I didn't believe that.

However, as time passed, I began to learn and grow as a person. Struggles and hardships in my life forced me to learn more, develop the desire to look deeper, and strive for more. My eyes opened to the world around me, and I finally burst out of the little bubble that I had been living in like an overgrown pimple. And it finally dawned on me...

I actually know **nothing...**

Or at the very least, I knew incredibly little. This bothered me, not just a little, but A LOT. I had a huge desire for knowledge, as it gave me a sense of control. When we don't understand things, we feel as though we have no control, and it freaks us out. And not knowing how my world around me "ticked" really freaked me out! I had to learn to *accept* that not knowing everything was OK, and to be honest, was actually better than knowing things.

Once you learn to accept the world around you for what it is, a mysterious and fantastic adventure without predictability or sense of control, it becomes much more fun to live in. Not only that, but you will also experience a feeling of freedom.

Once I finally learned to *"let go,"* life became less stressful and much more enjoyable. I was able to go with the flow and not worry so much about the little things in life that are so insignificant, but that we give so much of our focus to.

I would like to share a story about my friend, as it really put the world and my problems into perspective for me. I am not at liberty to discuss my friend's real name, but for this story we will call him Steve.

Steve had very harsh parents growing up. Both of his parents were extremely brutal and abusive. They stripped Steve's room of all of his belongings and locked him in there like a jail cell. There was mattress and a vent, and nothing else.

Solitary confinement is usually saved for the most wicked and despicable human beings in our society, those who steal, rape, and murder. Steve had to endure almost fifteen years of this torment without a single reason to deserve it. And to make matters worse, it was those who should have been there to love and protect him who were his wardens.

He spent day after day doing nothing. If he ever found a penny or a paperclip he was ecstatic! That is, until his father would find it, beat him, and then throw it away.

One day, he managed to smuggle a small rock into his cell (room). He would play with it non-stop. Eventually he got to the point where he could throw it off of one wall, have it skip around the room, and make it land perfectly back in his hand. If he heard his father's lumbering footsteps hastily approaching, he would quickly slide the rock into his air vent where he could retrieve it later. Eventually his father found that too, and punished Steve accordingly.

On another occasion, Steve's father obtained a dog whom Steve fell in love with. When Steve's father noticed his son's passion for the dog, he called Steve over and asked him about it.

Father: "You like this dog?"

Steve: "... Yeah?..."

Father: "Alright then."

His father then opened up the door and kicked the dog so hard that it would never return. For good measure, he even told Steve the next day that he had found the dog in the ditch, and that it had been run over by a car.

What kind of a man (I can't call him a father) would do this to his son?

There are many more stories about Steve and his father, some too gruesome to tell. However, the point is that Steve allowed me to see the world in a different light.

If you were to imagine talking with him, you might picture an angry, scarred young man, full of bitterness and hate. But actually, Steve is one of the most relaxed people I have ever met. Instead of letting his past define his future, he instead uses it to make his future better. Nothing fazes him, as he has dealt with things that were so much worse. He rarely gets angry or stresses out, and most of all never lets little things bug him. Personally, I believe he may want to eventually talk about his childhood abuse with a counselor. But for the time being, he says he is fine, and I have to believe him. If he is scarred deep down, he does a great job of hiding it, and he's currently living an extremely fulfilling life. I just hope that he is able to learn to cope before things get out of hand.

My perspective was forever changed after meeting Steve. I just couldn't stop thinking, *if he could deal with all of that, then how can I dwell on the insignificance of being hazed by a few college idiots?* I'm not taking ANYTHING away from my experience, or more importantly yours, as they are **very** real, **very** painful, and are nothing to take lightly. Instead, it simply allowed me to understand that life is a mindset. We cannot control *what* happens to us, but we CAN control *how* we react to it. It's all up to us. **Things are only as important as we make them.** I know some people who hate drinking water that's warm, and I know others who are thrilled to death to even have clean water to drink and would never even give a thought to the temperature. It's all a state of mind, but that doesn't make it easy.

What's the best way to learn this, you ask? Well, usually the best way to learn is to have something taken away from you. Only then can you truly appreciate what you had to begin with.

Take my buddy, for example. He had literally EVERYTHING taken away from him. His possessions, friends, clothes, and freedom were GONE! To some it might seem as though his entire childhood was stripped from him, and they'd be right. But if you were to ask *him*, he would say that it wasn't a waste at all. Of course he didn't enjoy the whole experience, but he found ways to *make* it enjoyable because he never once had the mindset of letting himself become the victim. He saw his circumstance and knew there was nothing he could do to fix it physically, so he did the only thing he could. He controlled how he *reacted* to it. This is an incredibly hard concept to master, but if you can manage to do it, I guarantee that your life will never be the same again.

It all comes down to the vantage point from which a person see things. One sees a cup as half empty, and the other sees the cup as half full. They are both right. However, due to their differences in mindset, one is able to look for the positive in a circumstance, while the other can only see the negative.

Try not to see the world as half empty. It really sucks. Just trust me and try to see it as half full. It's a lot better.

And if you are still struggling with the feeling that you "know it all," just try this.

Try to *listen* to what others have to say, even if you think (or KNOW) that they are wrong. At the very least, you won't come across as rude, and you will make them feel appreciated as a human being. But you may also come away with something that you didn't expect. This is only achieved through having an open mind, however, so try to "let go" and just see what others have to say. Ultimately, you will never know whether they are right or wrong until you listen to what they have to say and physically try their suggestions for yourself. If your doctor is telling you that the chemicals in your brain are out of whack and that you may need to take medication, at least listen with an open mind. *Maybe* he is right, or *maybe* he is wrong. You can't really say one way or the other until you test it out for yourself.

I would also recommend that if you are going to try something that affects your body, make sure it's prescribed by someone who actually KNOWS what they are talking about, preferably a licensed professional.

Also, if you do decide to try something, please **give it your full effort.** Doing things halfheartedly is a waste of your time and theirs. If something is worth doing, then it's worth doing well.

Find Meaning Beyond Life

This doesn't necessarily have to be spiritual, but for me it certainly was. It could simply mean allowing yourself to gain perspective on the "bigger picture"—to really contemplate why you are here and what legacy you want to leave behind.

One of my favorite quotes in history is this:

"History will be kind to me for I intend to write it." - Winston Churchill

Write your own history. It's truly an exciting concept to grasp. We have the ability to control our own destinies, and we can do virtually anything we set our minds to.

We can voice our opinions to the masses in ways that our ancestors could have never imagined. We can invent new possibilities, create masterpieces, discover true beauty, or simply discover inner peace. None of these is nobler than the other, and only YOU can truly know what your calling is. But I implore you to find it, to search your inner self, and to look deep into what makes you "tick."

I often go for long walks on abandoned trails, or bike through unexplored paths. I love the feeling of "getting lost" and allowing myself to discover new things. I find a certain serenity in being alone with my thoughts, and I often share them with my God. It allows me to take a step back from the chaos of life, and be able to truly recollect what is important to me and my life. It is not self-centered to be curious about your own internal desires, and it is truly amazing when you are able to find ones that are yours and yours alone— not influenced by society, or your friends, or even your parents, but *your own* passions for the life you want to live.

That is what it means to find meaning beyond life.

Pray

I believe prayer is extremely powerful. I realize that not everyone will share in my views, but if you are willing, I would love to lead you in a prayer that will invite God to work on your behalf.

Prayer gives us control over our lives. The devil came to steal, kill, and destroy, but luckily we have power over him through Jesus Christ. If we pray specifically that Satan no longer has the power to control us through depression and/or anxiety, then we can free ourselves from that oppression through Jesus Christ. It takes the away the devil's power, and forces him to relinquish his control over us and our minds.

If you are skeptical, then by all means feel free to skip over this, but I would highly encourage you to step outside of your comfort zone and give it a chance. You don't have to be in public. In fact, I would discourage it. Find a quiet place and try your best to focus on what you are saying, and believe in the words you are speaking about your life.

Think of it this way: if you try it, the worst that could happen is nothing. Yet, if this works the way I believe it will, then you'll be breaking Satan's power over you and finally taking back what is rightfully yours: peace.

So, if you are willing, repeat after me.

"Thank you, Jesus, for all that you have given me. Thank you so much for giving me power over my enemies through your mighty name. I pray that you will free me from the oppression of anxiety and depression that has hindered me from reaching my fullest potential. I know this is simply the enemy trying to keep me from the incredible destiny that awaits me. Please reveal yourself to me, and fill me with your love and mercy. Fill me with peace in my mind and joy in my soul. Thank you again for the power you have placed within me to control my destiny and future. I invite you to work on my behalf and fight for me in any and every circumstance. I pray these things in the name of Jesus Christ, Amen."

If you were able to step out of your comfort zone and pray just now, I am so incredibly proud of you. I know that wasn't easy, but the fact that you did it shows tremendous courage and strength of character. I truly hope God is able to reveal himself to you in a very real way, allow you peace of mind, and overflow your soul with joy! I know that he will.

If you were unable to recite this prayer for whatever reason, don't be ashamed. I realize that this is not for everyone and that I did not advertise this book as "spiritual." I only added this section because I felt that my entire being was being taken over by depression and anxiety, and that includes body, mind, soul, and spirit. Through the mercy of Jesus Christ, I was able to set my spirit free, and I only wished to share my experience with you. If this is not for you, or you are simply not comfortable with this for the time being, that is not a problem. You can always come back and repeat this prayer in the future if you feel led to.

It's OK To Be Sad

Understand that it is OK to be sad. We cry for a reason. It's not a mistake, or some freak accident. It allows us to process, to let go, and to move on.

Stuffing emotions and *pretending* to be happy is not healthy. This can lead to far worse problems down the road. Most commonly, it leads to "explosions" of emotions that harm either yourself or those around you.

Every day doesn't have to be the happiest day of your life. It's human to have ups and downs. One of my all-time favorite quotes comes from John Green, who said:

"That's the thing about pain. It demands to be felt."

I believe this is incredibly powerful. Pain is such a force that it DEMANDS to be felt. Trying to stop it would just be a waste of time, not to mention unhealthy.

The trouble starts when you start wallowing in your own grief long past the point of necessity, choosing pain over and over again. Doing that is unfair, not just to you but to those who care for you. You deserve to be happy, to enjoy life and experience it to the fullest. There is a difference between *feeling* pain and *choosing* pain. Feeling is natural, but choosing is not. A good way to tell if you are choosing pain is to look within yourself with an open mind.

Has something tragic occurred recently to cause this pain, such as someone close dying? A financial disappointment? A hard breakup?

These are all things that would cause *natural* pain, things that need to be grieved. It may take a day, a week, or a month–only you will be able to judge, but it WILL end. This pain won't be infinite. There will be a conclusion.

The key is learning the difference between pain that is natural, and that which is chosen. I wish I could tell you which type you are dealing with, but ultimately only YOU can know for sure.

I will say this: if you have been living in pain for more than a few months, then that is not natural. Anything that lasts longer than that is even less natural. Stop choosing pain, and start choosing life.

The Ultimate Challenge

Here's what it all boils down to in the end.

YOU MUST MAKE A CHOICE.

You have to physically, mentally, emotionally, and spiritually make the decision that you *want* to get better—that you *want* happiness and healing. You have to decide that you don't deserve the life you are currently living, and that you're going to do everything in your power to change it for the better. Commit yourself fully to the process, even when things get tough. And boy will they get tough! This journey will not be easy. There will be ups and downs, but if you learn to find strength in the struggle, then nothing can ever stop you!

The truth is, no one can make you do something you don't want to do, not your parents, your counselor, your favorite actor or celebrity, not even me. Only YOU can make that decision. It's your life, your body, your brain, your happiness, and ultimately, your journey. And it can't be won without fully committing yourself to the process.

I have seen it over and over and over again. The number one cause of a person's failure to change comes from a lack of personal commitment to the process. They may have initially thought this is was they wanted, but it wasn't. It was someone else in their life who wanted it *for* them. That doesn't work, since nobody else can make this journey for you! They can help you along, provide you comfort, and offer support. In fact, I believe it's vital that you have people who will do this. However, only YOU can truly change the outcome of your life and step into the incredible destiny that awaits you!

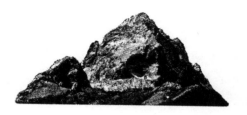

PART VI
How To Enjoy Life Again

"Perspective is everything. Even standing on Mount Everest means nothing to those who were born there. Only those who have had to suffer the treacherous climb can truly appreciate the beauty of their achievement."

Learn To Appreciate the "Little Things"

Life is full of beauty and wonder. It's easy to overlook the little things and take them for granted.

However, if we can find it in ourselves to rediscover their beauty, it can bring new meaning to our lives.

Take the time to appreciate simple things like flowers blooming, new-fallen snow, a refreshing cool breeze, or the warmth of the sun on your skin. Thousands of little moments pass us by daily, and each one is beautiful and wondrous in its own way. Learn to stop and take them in.

We live in a hurried time, always rushing from place to place. Just think, when was the last time you had a leisurely drive, where you weren't in a hurry and none of your fellow drivers bothered you?

Instead of rushing and stressing, if we can simply learn to *let go,* things become much more enjoyable. Imagine a world where you weren't constantly stressed about getting to this or that by a certain time. Imagine if you didn't mind getting caught in a little traffic, as long as you could enjoy the beauty around you. Imagine drifting off into deep thought and seeing it as a fantastic pleasure, rather than a complete waste of time. Imagine a world where you could just live freely, let go, and enjoy the little things.

Understand That You Are Stronger Now

Though I wouldn't wish depression on anyone, we who have experienced it are in an extremely privileged position. Let me explain.

We will most likely struggle with depression and anxiety more than others throughout our lives. This is just a fact that we don't have any control over. For whatever reason—chemical imbalances, life experiences, brain chemistry, whatever!—we are going to be more susceptible to fall back into our weaknesses. But here's the good news.

Since we were able to *understand* what was happening to us, *wanted* to change, and took the necessary *action* in order to do so, we are now better equipped than most people. We have the tools and resources in place, and the understanding and power to properly use them. We no longer have to sit in the back seat and let chance drive our lives. We now are in control of the wheel... and that is incredibly exciting!

You are now in complete control of yourself. There is no more worrying about "what if?"—you can respond and react accordingly to whatever life throws at you.

Being able to truly understand that *you* are in control is a huge anxiety reliever, because most cases of depression and anxiety disorders come from people being unable to control their circumstances. That was certainly the case for me. My first encounter was caused by a lack of control of my surroundings. I had no say in where I lived, and it terrified me. If I couldn't even control what country I lived in, how could I possibly control the much smaller aspects of my life? Well, here's the secret: **I couldn't.**

I couldn't control what happened to me, but I was always in control of how *I reacted*. In other words, I couldn't control anything except myself. I was always in charge of how I responded to each and every circumstance in my life, no matter how awful they may have been.

Trust the "Big Picture"

Having trust can be incredibly difficult when tough things happen. Some things in life just aren't fair and don't make sense. Mothers die during childbirth, innocent loved ones are killed in random car accidents, and wars hurt and kill thousands. There will always be things that you don't understand. Frankly, no one else does, either. Life isn't fair. So, how can you accept horrible things happening to great people? Here is my technique.

First, I want to warn you that you may not agree with what I am about to say. You may consider it foolish, and if so, I apologize. But this ideology has kept things in perspective for me in my darkest times, and therefore I wish to share it with you.

Trust. It's as simple as that.

"Trust what?" you may ask. Well, for me, I trust my Lord and savior Jesus Christ. I trust that he has a plan far greater than I could ever understand, and therefore I will let him carry it out without judgment. We ultimately have no idea how "this" affects "that." In the grand scheme of things, we are trying to solve a colossal puzzle while only being able to look at it through a drinking straw. We simply aren't capable of understanding it from our tiny vantage point. We don't have the proper perspective to understand what makes the world tick, so how can we possibly ask ourselves to solve its mysteries, such as bad things happening to good people?

If you aren't a believer in God, then please don't brush off this thinking as Christian nonsense. This is only MY personal philosophy. No Christian leader, pastor, or minister taught it to me. I found this during my darkest time, struggling to find any meaning in life when I was all alone at university. I went for countless long walks, spending two hours or more deep in thought each time. I weighed every possible outcome I could think of for why things happen to people... and ultimately I couldn't come up with anything. That's when I finally realized it's all right not to know.

Living in the information era causes a massive desire to want to know and understand everything. If we don't know something, we simply Google the phrase, and we are given instant information. This gives us peace, because the unknown scares us. So, what do we do when there is no answer—when we can't just hop on Wikipedia and find exactly what we are looking for? Well, the answer is that we have to trust in the big picture.

Whether you believe in a God or not, you have to trust that things happen for a reason. Not only that, but you have to be OK with not always knowing what that reason is.

I look at it like this. We make thousands of choices every day—small choices that we don't even think about. But just imagine how we leave our footprint on the world with each small decision we make.

For example, let's say you just finished parking at the grocery store. You turn off your car, open the door, and step outside. The air is warm, and the sun feels amazing on your cold skin. As you walk toward the grocery store, you pass a man who looks at you for a split second. You don't even notice him. You keep walking.

Stop here and think... how could your action have affected that man's future? (This is simply an example, but it isn't so far-fetched.)

Let's say that, on this particular day, this man is feeling extremely lonely. In fact, he has been feeling lonely for weeks. He struggles with anxiety and depression, and he desperately seeks the approval of others. He is so insecure that he constantly lets others' opinions of him control his opinion of himself.

He desperately seeks approval and belonging from all those he encounters. He can't help it—he doesn't even realize he's doing it.

He's at the grocery store buying milk, but in reality, he just wanted to be around other people for a little while. He takes every opportunity to make that happen. He spends extra time strolling around, browsing items he doesn't even remotely need or want, all in an attempt to avoid going back to his lonely apartment.

Finally, the time comes when he must leave, and he buys his milk through the self-checkout. Though he loves to be around people, he is so insecure that even talking to a cashier sends shivers down his spine. He walks timidly out of the shade of the grocery store and into the blaze of sunlight outside. He notices a strong, confident man walking toward him and immediately admires him. He isn't even sure what is drawing him towards this stranger. Perhaps it's his clothing, his hairstyle, or maybe his car.

No, it's his confidence. The stranger is secure in who he is, and that's something our guy doesn't have.

In an involuntary request for approval, our guy makes every effort to make eye contact and secure this stranger's blessing. He goes out of his way to make the subtle contact happen, while also trying to avoid being too obvious or appearing desperate. He strains his neck as he passes, hoping the stranger will turn at the last second, but he doesn't. Our guy is mortified.

The stranger, who he grew to admire so greatly in mere seconds, completely ignores him. Our guy feels like he's so pathetic that he doesn't even exist in the stranger's world. He thinks, "If this guy doesn't even have the desire to look at me and give me a quick smile of approval, then why am I here?"

Our guy reflects on this encounter all day, replaying it over and over again in his head. As a result, this simple, meaningless act controls the rest of his day. He is so engrossed in his own thoughts that he doesn't even realize that he has drifted into oncoming traffic. By the time he hears the horn blaring and is snapped back into reality, it is too late. He slams head on into a minivan driven by a mother taking her two sons home from soccer practice.

The mother is killed on impact. The eldest son

sustains serious brain swelling and ends up in critical condition. The doctors don't know if he will ever wake up from his coma. The youngest son suffers only a minor break to his arm, along with some other scrapes and bruises. He will make a full recovery from his injuries, but the trauma from the accident, the death of his mother, and possibly the loss of his older brother, will haunt him the rest of his life. He and his father will try to move on somehow, with half of their hearts missing.

What's your reaction to my hypothetical story? Are you thinking that this is a freak accident, something that will never happen? You're probably right, but we don't know for sure. That's my point. We just don't know. We have absolutely no idea how even our smallest actions affect the grand scheme of life.

In this example, it definitely wasn't the stranger's fault for simply not noticing the lonely man leaving the grocery store. And it certainly was not the fault of the poor family, who did nothing to deserve this fate. However, it also wasn't the fault of the lonely man. He had no intention of harming anyone and wasn't even doing anything illegal at the time. However, for whatever reason, a series of unfortunate occurrences caused this event to take place.

Perhaps if the stranger had simply smiled at him, the lonely man would have felt appreciated, and none of this would have happened. Perhaps if he had simply gotten the help he needed beforehand, such as seeing a counselor or talking with loved ones, then he wouldn't have been so distracted. Or even if the mother had simply left 10 seconds earlier or 10 seconds later, no accident would have taken place. It was nobody's *fault,* yet it still happened... so how do we explain it?

Put simply, we can't. Shit happens (excuse the language, but it's true). It's a part of life. We can't control it or understand it. We can only react to it. However, if we learn to trust in the big picture, then we won't feel such a need to understand it. In turn, we'll allow ourselves to live a life of freedom.

If you still have a problem with my story, thinking it was too far-fetched, don't. The lonely man was modeled after me. Although luckily I didn't have my license during my darkest days, it isn't a stretch to imagine that I might have caused an accident if I had.

I lived like that for years, desperately seeking the approval of others, and putting my own thoughts into their heads if they didn't respond how I had hoped—or even if they did respond. It caused me incredible anxiety and nearly drove me mad. I was always reading too much into people's actions or body language and assuming the worst. It was a result of my immense insecurity and my overactive brain. That was a deadly combination for me and nearly drove me insane. If I'd had my license at the time, who knows what might have happened. That's exactly my point: *who knows?*

Instead of trying to understand *why* things happen, just trust that they are happening for a reason. Who knows whether that encounter led the lonely man to devote his life to helping the homeless or feeding orphans? Perhaps the young boy in the car became a motivational speaker later in life, used his own tragedy to help others get through their own, and possibly saved hundreds of lives. Or perhaps nothing so dramatic happened at all. Maybe the accident caused small internal changes in both the lonely man and the young boy that would affect how they treated others for the rest of their lives. These small changes can literally change the world, just not in a rapid or obvious way. But if you track the ripple effect of ALL of the encounters those two people will have in their lifetimes, you cannot say that this unfair and tragic event didn't change the world in some way. It is up to us to determine whether that change will be for the better or worse.

Your Lowest Valley Becomes Your Highest Peak!

I know I have used this quote already, but it's worth hearing again: *"You never know happy unless you've known sad."* I truly believe that you can only experience peaks as high as the depth of your lowest valley. When you were at your absolute worst—when you had hit rock bottom, everything was going wrong, and you had no idea what your purpose on this earth was anymore—you sunk to a depth that is unknown to many. As extreme a low as that was... you can now experience that intensity of happiness.

Many of the most successful and influential people in our world had to go through all kinds of hardships and failures to get where they are. If you have already gone through an extremely tough stretch, or if you're in one now, you can be sure that what you're learning will make you a stronger person and prepare you for a better future.

I personally have a new lease on life after coming out of my last episode of depression. I am more patient and kind. Above all else, I no longer take things for granted. Any day that I wake up and don't feel horrible is a good day! I'm so grateful for each one! After being at such a low place for such a long time, I can now appreciate "average" days as spectacular ones!

I no longer take my parents' love for me for granted, and what used to drive me nuts about them, I now cherish. Once I learned what it felt like to "lose" them, I discovered how much I really care, and how insignificant my issues with them really were.

Another thing that I no longer take for granted is the ability to live without constant anxiety. I suffered with that for months, and it's shown me how blessed we are to simply not be in pain all the time. It's not just the absence of anxiety, either. The vast majority of us are not living with any diseases or injuries that cause us daily pain, and I think we sometimes forget how fortunate we are!

If you are someone who lives in constant pain, I

commend you. You are truly a hero in my eyes, and I'm certain that you were created with a special purpose in life! I don't know for sure, but my guess is that you probably have the best perspective on life out of all of us. You aren't easily caught up in the latest trends, and most likely aren't influenced by media and peer pressure. You keep the big picture in mind and don't forget what it truly important in life. Don't ever let your pain get the best of you, no matter how hard it gets! Let it drive and fuel you to greatness instead. Turn your weakness into strength. I won't lie and say that it's easy, or even that I know what it's truly like. But I know that you were created with a special purpose, and my greatest desire would be to witness you achieve it! So shoot for the stars and don't hold anything back. You rock!

If the above paragraph didn't apply to you, don't think you can't use it as motivation. Read it again, and realize just how fortunate you are to not have to deal with pain. Though I believe that those who do are destined for greatness, that doesn't mean it won't be incredibly hard for them. Pain sucks. So if you are fortunate enough to live the majority of your life without it, don't take that for granted!

I know that I talk a lot about perspective and the "big picture," but that's only because it's so essential to preventing yourself from getting caught up in the meaningless stuff, and living the most fulfilled life that you can!

Keep this quote in mind.

"Only if you have been in the deepest valley, can you ever know how magnificent it is to be on the highest mountain."

- Richard Nixon

Standing on Everest means nothing if you were born there. The beauty is in the journey. A sense of accomplishment cannot be obtained by outcomes alone, but rather by the process in which the outcomes are achieved. The deeper your valley is, the more magnificent the summit will be!

We Can Help Others in Similar Situations

Once we have taken massive action in our own lives, and changed the course of them for the better, we can then use the skills we learned along the way to help other people who need it. There are countless people who are struggling with the same or similar things that we did. Since we have been there, we can relate better than anyone else possibly can! Our advice and encouragement carries more weight than words from someone who has only knowledge but no experience. You can read about something all you want, but if you have never personally experienced it, then how could you ever call yourself an expert? So since we *have* been through so much, we are experts. And it would be a travesty not to share what we have learned and help out those who are struggling to find direction!

That is the main vision behind this book. I hope that by sharing my story and my strategies for overcoming the hardships in my life, I can help those who may be without hope—those who don't have direction, or just need a little boost to keep going.

Again, I am no doctor. I don't have a university

degree or a family of my own yet. I'm just a kid who has experienced more than most, and wants to share his experiences with those who wish to hear them. I've seen this disease of depression spread like wildfire around me, especially in those my age. Therefore, I felt it to be my duty to help in the only way that I could: by sharing my story. If I can impact one life in writing this book, then it will all be worth it.

If you've read this book in its entirety, I want to thank you from the bottom of my heart. It wasn't easy to share my experiences, but I know that they have the power to help others. If you know someone who is struggling and believe this book could somehow benefit them, then please share it. That was the whole point in writing it.

If you *are* someone who is struggling, then I truly hope you were able to find some peace through reading my story. You *are* going to make it through this, and I'm not just saying that.

In fact, I feel so passionate about this topic that I want you to be able to reach out to me if you desire. So please, if you want someone to talk to or have any questions that you want answered privately, PLEASE contact me at jacobreimer@depressionmybattle.com. I will do my best to respond to you as quickly as I possibly can, and if this email is still public when you are reading, then I am still actively responding personally.

Your life is incredibly special, and I want you to see it the way that I do.

128

ABOUT THE AUTHOR

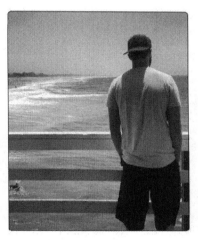

I live a pretty extraordinarily normal life. I currently reside in beautiful British Columbia, Canada, with my amazing family, whom I love. I am currently a full-time author at the age of 20, and I am LOVING every minute of it.

While I may be young in age, I believe my experiences and incredible adventures give me a unique perspective —a point of view you couldn't get from anyone else.

I try to live every day as if it were my last, allowing myself to fully experience the highs and lows of each and every day. I refuse to let myself get hung up on insignificant events, and instead choose to respond with positivity, optimism, and love.

If you enjoyed my book, I strongly encourage you to join my author newsletter. I promise I won't spam your inbox, but will just give you a heads up on new book releases (and possibly better deals!). If that is something that interests you, then you can sign up at www.DepressionMyBattle.com (It's 100% free.) If not, then no worries.

Thank you so much and have a great day!

ACKNOWLEDGEMENTS

As I close this book, I thought it would be improper if I didn't thank those who helped me along the way.

First and foremost, I would like to thank my wonderful family. Without their constant love and support, I wouldn't be here right now.

In addition to them, I would also like to thank my dear friends. You were there for me when all else were absent, and you will never understand how much that means to me.

I would also like to thank Stefan Plynarimos, without whom I would have never gotten into writing or self publishing.

Last but not least, I would like to thank my editor Cara Stein. I can truly say that she fought alongside me in the creation of this book. Without you, this book would be but a shadow of what it is today, and for that I thank you Cara. You truly are an inspiration to me.

In fact, I would like to show my gratitude by giving

others the opportunity to work with you if they so please. Cara is truly a professional in all aspects of the word, but even more so she truly CARES about not just the book... but what it has to say.

If you would like to get in contact with Cara you can do so at www.bookcompletion.com. She is prolific in editing, book cover design, and preparing books for Kindle and print.' I promise you will not regret it.

Thank you once again for reading this book. I truly hope it was able to help you along in your journey, and believe me when I say... the best is yet to come!

Made in the USA
Lexington, KY
18 April 2017